Medical Research
Scientific Writing and Publishing

Akmal El-Mazny

CONTENTS

INTRODUCTION	1
CHAPTER I: RESEARCH MANAGEMENT	2
I- RESEARCH PROCESS	3
II- RESEARCH PRINCIPLES	9
CHAPTER II: SCIENTIFIC WRITING	12
I- TITLE	17
II- ABSTRACT	18
III- INTRODUCTION	20
IV- MATERIALS AND METHODS	22
1- Study Design	23
Introduction to Evidence-Based Medicine	29
2- Setting	35
3- Participants	36
4- Interventions	39
5- Follow-up	40
6- Outcome Measures	43
7- Statistical Analysis	44
Introduction to Biomedical Statistics	45
V- RESULTS	74
VI- DISCUSSION	77
VII- REFERENCES	81
CHAPTER III: RESEARCH PUBLISHING	87
I- UNIFORM REQUIREMENTS	89
II- REVIEW PROCESS	91
REFERENCES	100

INTRODUCTION

Scientific writing and publishing marks the endpoint of medical research that has been performed, completed, reviewed and accepted, and complements teaching and training, clinical service and patient care.

This book instructs, in a very clear style, the guidelines authors should follow in order to improve the quality of their scientific papers.

Chapter I provides an overview on the application and implementation of internationally accepted principles for research practice.

Chapter II presents in details all the necessary steps of research design and scientific writing; including an essential introduction to evidence-based medicine and biomedical statistics.

Chapter III describes the uniform requirements of biomedical journals as well as the editorial and review processes for research publishing.

Everything is easy when you know how – I hope that this book will provide the "know how" for all researchers, academicians and health-care professionals.

CHAPTER I:

RESEARCH MANAGEMENT

This chapter outlines WHO key activities and principles involved in the good clinical research practice (GCP).

Multiple parties are responsible for the success of these activities; the investigators, sponsors, ethics committees, and regulatory authorities.

The principles of GCP should generally apply to all clinical research involving human subjects:

- Studies of a physiological, biochemical, or pathological process, or of the response to a specific intervention – whether physical, chemical, or psychological – in healthy subjects or in patients;
- Controlled studies of diagnostic, preventive or therapeutic measures, designed to demonstrate a specific generalizable response to these measures against a background of individual biological variation;
- Studies designed to determine the consequences for individuals and communities of specific preventive or therapeutic measures;
- Studies concerning human health-related behavior in a variety of circumstances and environments;
- Studies that employ either observation or physical, chemical, or psychological intervention.

I- RESEARCH PROCESS

1. Trial Protocol:

Integral to protocol development are the concepts of risk identification, study design and control groups, and statistical methodology.

2. Standard Operating Procedures (SOPs):

– Developing and updating the protocol, investigator's brochure, case report forms (CRFs), and other study-related documents;

– Supplies procurement, shipping, handling, and accounting for all supplies of the investigational product;

– Standardizing the activities of sponsors and study personnel (e.g. review of adverse event reports by medical experts; data analysis by statisticians);

– Standardizing the activities of clinical investigators to ensure that trial data is accurately captured;

– Monitoring, to ensure that processes are consistently followed and activities are consistently documented;

– Auditing, to determine whether monitoring is being appropriately carried out and the systems for quality control are operational and effective.

3. Support Systems and Tools:

– Diagnostic or laboratory equipment required by the study protocol, and procedures/schedules for servicing the equipment according to the manufacturer's specifications;

– Computer systems (hardware and software) to be used in the clinical trial (e.g. statistical or other software, electronic patient diaries, coding of personal data), and software validation systems, as needed;

– Facsimile or other communications equipment to facilitate reporting of serious adverse events;

– Information and training tools for clinical investigators and site personnel.

4. Trial-related Documents:

– Investigator's brochure;

– Checklists to identify and document the required steps for each of the various clinical trial activities (e.g. investigator selection, approvals and clearances, monitoring, adverse event reporting and evaluation, analysis of interim data);

– Investigational supplies accountability forms to document the amount and source of investigational product shipped and received, the amount dispensed to subjects, and the return/destruction, as appropriate, of any unused product;

– Signature logs and other forms to document by whom activities are completed, when, and the sequence in which they are carried out;

– Case report forms (CRFs) for each scheduled study visit to capture all of the necessary data collected from and reported for each subject;

– Informed consent documents;

– Adverse event or safety reporting forms;

– Administrative forms to track research funds and expenses;

– Forms to disclose information about the investigator's interests in the product under study, in accordance with national regulations.

5. Trial Sites, Investigators and Personnel:

Clinical investigators must be qualified and have sufficient resources and appropriately trained staff to conduct the investigation and be knowledgeable of the national setting and circumstances of the site and study population(s).

6. Ethics Committee Review:

Studies must be reviewed and receive approval/favorable opinion from an Independent Ethics Committee (IEC)/Institutional Review Board (IRB) prior to enrollment of study subjects.

7. Review by Regulatory Authorities:

Studies must undergo review by regulatory authorities for use of the investigational product or intervention in human subjects and to ensure that the study is appropriately designed to meet its stated objectives, according to national/regional/local law and regulations.

8. Enrollment of Subjects into the Study:

The clinical investigator has primary responsibility for recruiting subjects, ensuring that only eligible subjects are enrolled in the study, and obtaining and documenting the informed consent of each subject.

9. The Investigational Product(s):

Quality of the investigational product is assured by compliance with Good Manufacturing Practice (GMP) and by handling and storing the product according to the manufacturing specifications and the study protocol.

10. Trial Data Acquisition:

Study records documenting each trial-related activity provide critical verification that the study has been carried out in compliance with the protocol.

11. Safety Management:

Although all parties who oversee or conduct clinical research have a role/responsibility for the safety of the study subjects, the clinical investigator has primary responsibility for alerting the sponsor and the IEC/IRB to adverse events, particularly serious or life-threatening unanticipated events, observed during the course of the research.

12. Monitoring the Trial:

The sponsor-investigator should determine the appropriate extent and nature of monitoring based on the objective, purpose, design, complexity, size, blinding, and endpoints of the trial, and the risks posed by the investigational product.

13. Managing Trial Data:

− Data acquisition;
− Confidentiality of data/data privacy;
− Electronic data capture (if applicable);
− Data management training for investigators and staff;
− Completion of CRFs and other trial-related documents, and procedures for correcting errors in such documents;
− Coding/terminology for adverse events, medication, medical histories;
− Safety data management and reporting;

- Data entry and data processing (including laboratory and external data);
- Database closure;
- Database validation;
- Secure, efficient, and accessible data storage;
- Data quality measurement (i.e. how reliable are the data) and quality assurance;
- Management of vendors (e.g. CROs, pharmacies, laboratories, software suppliers, off-site storage) that participate directly or indirectly in managing trial data and materials.

14. Quality Assurance:

Quality assurance (QA) verifies through systematic, independent audits that existing quality control systems (e.g. study monitoring; data management systems) are working and effective.

15. Reporting the Trial:

- A description of the ethical aspects of the study (e.g. confirmation that the study was conducted in accordance with basic ethical principles);
- A description of the administrative structure of the study (i.e. identification and qualifications of investigators/sites/other facilities);
- An introduction that explains the critical features and context of the study (e.g. rationale and aims, target population, treatment duration, primary endpoints);
- A summary of the study objectives;
- A description of the overall study design and plan;
- A description of any protocol amendments;

− An accounting of all subjects who participated in the study, including all important deviations from inclusion/exclusion criteria and a description of subjects who discontinued after enrollment;

− An accounting of protocol violations;

− A discussion of any interim analyses;

− An efficacy evaluation, including specific descriptions of subjects who were included in each efficacy analysis and listing of all subjects who were excluded from the efficacy analysis and the reasons for such exclusion;

− A safety evaluation, including extent of exposure, common adverse events and laboratory test changes, and serious or unanticipated or other significant adverse events including evaluation of subjects who left the study prematurely because of an adverse event or who died;

− A discussion and overall conclusions regarding the efficacy and safety results and the relationship of risks and benefits;

− Tables, figures, and graphs that visually summarize the important results or to clarify results that are not easily understood;

− A reference list.

II- Research Principles

Principle 1:

Research involving humans should be scientifically sound and conducted in accordance with basic ethical principles, which have their origin in the Declaration of Helsinki. Three basic ethical principles of equal importance, namely respect for persons, beneficence, and justice, permeate all other GCP principles.

Principle 2:

Research involving humans should be scientifically justified and described in a clear, detailed protocol.

Principle 3:

Before research involving humans is initiated, foreseeable risks and discomforts and any anticipated benefit(s) for the individual research subject and society should be identified. Research of investigational products or procedures should be supported by adequate non-clinical and, when applicable, clinical information.

Principle 4:

Research involving humans should be initiated only if the anticipated benefit(s) for the individual research subject and society clearly outweigh the risks. Although the benefit of the results of the trial to science and society should be taken into account, the most important considerations are those related to the rights, safety, and well-being of the research subjects.

Principle 5:

Research involving humans should receive independent ethics committee/institutional review board (IEC/IRB) approval/favorable opinion prior to initiation.

Principle 6:

Research involving humans should be conducted in compliance with the approved protocol.

Principle 7:

Freely given informed consent should be obtained from every subject prior to research participation in accordance with national culture(s) and requirements.

Principle 8:

Research involving humans should be continued only if the benefit-risk profile remains favorable.

Principle 9:

Qualified and duly licensed medical personnel (i.e. physician or, when appropriate, dentist) should be responsible for the medical care of research subjects, and for any medical decision(s) made on their behalf.

Principle 10:

Each individual involved in conducting a trial should be qualified by education, training, and experience to perform his or her respective task(s) and currently licensed to do so, where required.

Principle 11:

All clinical trial information should be recorded, handled, and stored in a way that allows its accurate reporting, interpretation, and verification.

Principle 12:

The confidentiality of records that could identify subjects should be protected, respecting the privacy and confidentiality rules in accordance with the applicable regulatory requirement(s).

Principle 13:

Investigational products should be manufactured, handled, and stored in accordance with applicable Good Manufacturing Practice (GMP) and should be used in accordance with the approved protocol.

Principle 14:

Systems with procedures that assure the quality of every aspect of the trial should be implemented.

CHAPTER II:

SCIENTIFIC WRITING

There are three key stages for "Effective scientific Writing" that should go sequentially and not simultaneously:

− Plan,

− Execute, and

− Polish.

Effective scientific writing is composed not only of valid scientific content, but also of good structure and effective style.

A well written scientific paper explains the scientist's motivation for doing an experiment, the experimental design and execution, and the meaning of the results.

There are general guidelines, which means that anybody can improve their scientific writing skills by learning them.

Some of the guidelines apply to all writing, not just scientific writing, and these are mostly aimed at improving clarity.

Other guidelines are specific to writing articles for scientific journals and are often concerned with the structure of the article.

In short, the writing can be just as challenging as the research!

Why are you writing?

Be realistic about trying to get your work published.

Your article must be suitable for the journal, and you should be prepared to make revisions.

You must work out why you are writing an article:
– You have made a minor, but very interesting, observation.
– You have made a useful advance.
– You are putting published information into a new context.
– You are synthesizing information in a novel way that will be of interest to others.

Your reasons must guide how you write and your choice of journal.

Writing Skills:

Writing is all about communication: you are telling people about your ideas and results.

Grab the reader's attention – science writing does not have to be boring!

There are often several good ways to say the same thing, not one "correct" way, so use the style that is easiest for you.

Write Clearly:

- Use simple language; you will not be there to explain to the reader what you mean.

- If you have to read a sentence again in order to understand it, rewrite it.

- Better still; give your work to others to read to see if it makes sense to them.

- Start with generalities and then move towards more specific ideas.

- Transmit one message per sentence, and avoid one sentence paragraph.

- Write coherent paragraphs (one idea per paragraph); there should be an obvious logical connection between paragraphs.

- Use simple and common words, avoid "big" words e.g. sacrifice – kill, utilize – use, terminate – end etc…

- Use 1st person, use active voice: "We collected data"; not "Data were collected"…

- Avoid special terms or abbreviations whenever you can; if you must use an abbreviation, write it out when it occurs the first time.

- Do not use contractions: e.g. can't, don't.

Write Concisely:

- Write with an economy of words.

- This keeps your writing from being swamped with unnecessary words.

- Keep sentences short: replace "based upon the fact that" and "for the purpose of" with "because" and "to"; "He advanced an argument for the proposition that…" vs. "He argued that…"

- All journals have strict word limits!

Write Correctly:

- Each sentence should give you all the information you need.
- Use correct tense of verbs, correct use of measurements, as well as correct spelling and grammar.
- Use the same definitions throughout – if you introduce a definition in the methods, use the same term in the results and discussion.
- Check your references.
- Get help for English language editing.

Writing Style:

Voice:

Basically, if the subject of a sentence performs the action, the sentence is in active voice.

The sentence is in passive voice if the subject of the sentence receives the action.

General Style: Use active voice.

Person:

Use first-person pronouns (I, we) to denote agents of action, which avoids wordiness and confusion.

General Style: Use first person.

Tense:

Scientific writing uses two major tenses: present and past.

Here are the general rules:

− Established information: present tense.

− Methods and Results sections: past tense.

− Presentation of data: present tense.

− Attribution of information (e.g., someone else's work): past tense.

Structure of Scientific Paper:

− Title.

− Abstract.

− Introduction: What question was asked?

− Material and methods: How was it studied?

− Results: What was found?

− Discussion: What do the findings mean?

− References.

I- TITLE

The title is a major determinant whether your paper will be found and whether people will be attracted enough to read it.

It is the only aspect that appears in tables of contents and in many data bases that are used to search for relevant publications.

Characteristics:
- Short and succinct.
- Reflects the main focus of the paper.
- Contains enough relevant key words "search terms".

Style:
- Descriptive Style: States the focus of the study.
- Conclusion Style: Provides a very brief summary of what the authors found.

Main elements:
- The name of the disease studied,
- The particular aspect or system studied, and
- The variable(s) manipulated.

The running title:
A second more brief title will appear as a header on every other page of the printed article.

II- **ABSTRACT**

It is the most or only read part and should be the most polished as it appears in the biomedical databases and is the basis for judgment by editors, assessors and readers.

Characteristics:

— Concise (150-250 words).

— Brief summary of core points.

— Well known abbreviations.

— Should stand alone.

— Required by most journals to be structured.

Style:

— Make your abstract intelligible as much as possible to a general readership.

— Indicate the value of your work.

— Puts your work into context and presents your conclusions.

— Tells us what you did.

— Tells us what you found out.

— Doesn't provide statistics.

— Clearly states the implications of your findings.

— Must not go beyond the maximum number of words asked for by the journal.

— Doesn't include references.

The abstract is written as a mini-paper and it usually contains the following information in this order:

- Introduction/objectives: A few sentences to provide background information on the problem you have investigated.
- Methods: The techniques you used.
- Results: The major results you present in the paper including quantitative information when possible.
- Conclusion: Interpretation of the results.

Keywords

These are what people use when searching for articles in literature indexes.

They should be quite specific to your topic.

III- INTRODUCTION

Introduction is meant to introduce the reader to your research and to discuss the results and conclusions of previously published studies, to help explain why the current study is of scientific interest.

You need to grab the reader's attention and convince him that it is worth reading the rest of the paper.

The introduction is organized to move from general information to specific information.

This background must be summarized succinctly; limit the introduction to studies that relate directly to the present study.

The research question should be Feasible, Interesting, Novel, Ethical, and Relevant (FINER).

The introduction should not be too long, or it will be swamped with unnecessary information and mislead the reader.

The introduction itself should have a logical structure to it and should flow from paragraph to paragraph.

It is very important to remember that the introduction (and indeed the whole paper) should be prepared with the reader in mind.

This means that you should not just download your view and information, but actually construct the introduction so that it follows a logical story and explains necessary things to the reader.

The first paragraph should introduce some general aspect of the study.

The second paragraph can go on to more specific issues, perhaps those particularly relevant to your study.

Subsequent paragraphs may add more detail or outline particular problems.

The final paragraph should focus in on the objectives of your study; this will be a good transition to the next section of the article which is the methods.

It is important to cite sources in the introduction section of your paper as evidence of the claims you are making.

While writing, try to answer these questions:
– Why did you perform the study?
– What gap of knowledge did you attempt to fill?
– What controversy did you try to resolve?

IV- MATERIALS AND METHODS

It provides information on what was used and what was done to study the research question.

Although materials (subjects) and methods section may be one of the easiest written parts of the research and may be the first part to be written, yet it needs much skill, it is the first part to be appraised usually and it is usually the main cause for absolute rejection of the work.

The objectives of materials and methods section are:
− The knowledgeable reader will believe that you are a competent and qualified investigator.
− Other researchers can reproduce your research exactly as you did.

In general, scientific writing is not an easy job, so start writing simple sentences, then rearrange in a more elaborate manner till reaching the satisfactory form. Writing is in the past tense.

The basic components of subjects and methods are:
1. Study Design.
2. Setting.
3. Participants (subjects, patients, cases).
4. Interventions.
5. Follow-up.
6. Outcome measures.
7. Statistical analysis.

1- *Study Design*

It is basic for any researcher to be aware by the different study designs and should always determine the design of the study.

Research can be classified into two main categories:
- Descriptive research and
- Comparative (analytical) research.

The major difference between the two categories is the absence of a control group in descriptive research and the presence of a control group in comparative research.

Descriptive Research:

Deals with only one group of patients so comparisons cannot be done and final solid conclusions cannot be drawn from.

Case Report:

A descriptive research that reports a rare or an unusual disease or a disorder usually in a single patient.

Case Series:

A research that reports the natural history of a disease or disorder in a group of patients or the outcome of a certain intervention or exposure in a group of patients.

Characteristics of descriptive research:

− No control group.

− Suitable for newly discovered phenomena.

− Does not fulfill the validity criteria.

− Least evidence.

Comparative (Analytical) Research:

Compares between two or more groups, and is further subdivided into two main categories: experimental and observational studies.

While observational studies can be subjected to many types of bias by its nature, experimental studies especially randomized controlled trials are the least design liable to bias.

Thus, randomized controlled trials are the corner stone of EBM and the design that gives the best evidence.

Experimental Studies:

The investigators assign the intervention to both the experimental and the control groups.

Simply they, the investigators, are the ones who decide "who takes what?" e.g. the intervention or the placebo.

Randomized Controlled Trial (RCT):

The investigators assign the intervention to both the experimental and the control groups by chance (at random).

Characteristics of RCT:

- True experiment with best evidence.
- Used mainly in therapeutic evaluation.
- Control group ensures specificity of treatment effect.
- Randomization ensures balanced groups (confounders).
- Blinding ensures patient and observer bias.
- Relatively difficult and costly.
- Ethical issues.

Non-Randomized Controlled Trial (Non-RCT):

The investigators did not use random assignment of the intervention to the experimental and the control groups.

Observational Studies:

According to their relation to time, observational studies are further sub-classified into cohort, case-control, and cross sectional studies.

Cohort Study:

One group is exposed to a certain exposure and the other (control group) is not or is exposed to the comparison exposure, and both groups are followed up forward in time till the occurrence of the outcome.

Characteristics of cohort study:

- The best alternative to RCT.

- Can establish cause effect relationship.

- Study multiple risk factors and outcomes.

- No ethical issues.

- No randomization.

- Time consuming and expensive.

- Not suitable for rare or long term outcomes.

Case-Control Study:

A research that starts with the outcome (a group of patients having a certain disease and another disease-free control group) and looks backward in time (either by recalling the history of exposure or looking for the exposure in the hospital records).

Characteristics of case-control study:

- Suitable for rare or long term outcomes.

- Easy, cheap and no ethical issues.

- No randomization.

- No control on confounders.

- Recall bias.

Cross-Sectional Study:

A research that compares between two groups in the same moment in time without either backward recall or forward follow-up.

Characteristics of cross-sectional study:

− Suitable to study the value of diagnostic tests.

− No follow-up.

− Fast and inexpensive.

− Gives prevalence of a disease or risk factor.

− Cannot measure incidence.

− Cannot establish a causal relationship.

− Limited information about prognosis.

The following chart shows the basic study design types:

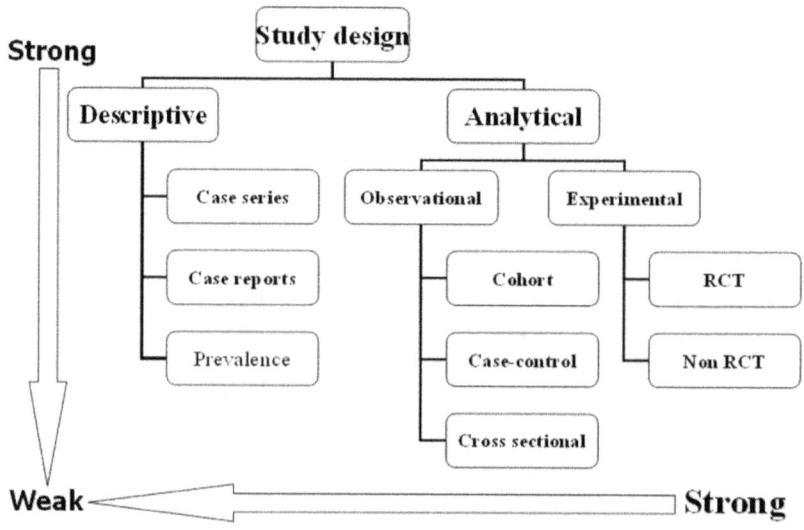

Study Design

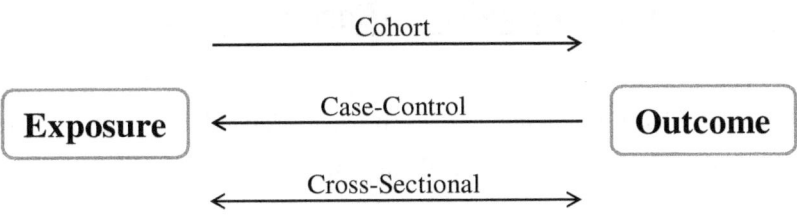

Observational Studies

General rules:

— Try to construct clear, simple, short, informative sentences.

— A simple design may be mentioned at the end of the introduction and the methodology starts with describing the subjects.

— Mention whether your data are primary or secondary data; secondary data are data collected for a different purpose than your study.

— If you performed multi-step designs, you should mention clearly.

Introduction to Evidence-Based Medicine:

Evidence-Based Medicine (EBM) is a problem-solving approach for questions that arise during clinical practice.

It is defined as "the integration of best research evidence with clinical expertise and patient values in direct patient care". *David Sackett*

Practicing EBM includes the following steps (5 As Model):

1. Assessment of the Patient:

Assessment of the patient is done by:
- History taking,
- Examination and
- Investigations.

2. Asking Clinical Questions:

Asking clinical question is to convert the patient's problems into clinical questions in a specific format (PICO format) where:
- P is the problem of the patient,
- I is the intervention or exposure,
- C is the comparison intervention or exposure, and
- O is the outcome the patient looks for (patient-oriented outcome).

3. Acquiring the Best Available Evidence:

Generally, there are three distinct, but interdependent, areas of EBM for finding the best answer (evidence) for the clinical questions generated:

The first is to treat individual patients by treatments supported in the most scientifically valid medical literature; thus, medical practitioners would select treatment options for specific cases based on the best research for each patient they treat.

The second area is the systematic review of medical literature to evaluate the best studies on specific topics; this process can be human-centered, as in a journal club, or technical, using computer programs and information techniques such as data mining.

Finally, EBM can be understood as a medical "movement" in which advocates work to popularize the method and usefulness of the practice in the public, patient communities, educational institutions, and continuing education of practicing professionals.

4. Appraisal of the Evidence:

Whenever one searches for evidence, he should start looking for the best available one which is obtained from (in descending order of importance):

- Systematic reviews and meta-analysis.

- Randomized controlled studies.

- Non-randomized controlled studies.

- Cohort studies.

- Case control studies.

- Case series.

- Case reports.

- Opinions of experts or respected authorities.

- Animal research and in-vitro studies.

The easiest way for a clinician is to start practicing EBM as an evidence "replicator" who follow evidence-based clinical guidelines, so he does not have to go into steps 3 and 4 (searching and appraising).

Another way of practicing EBM is to be an evidence "user" who can search for readily pre-appraised evidence directly without going into step 4 (appraising).

But with time and practice clinicians would face problems in which there is no readily made evidence to replicate or use; in such circumstances a clinician has to do critical appraisal and practice as an evidence "doer".

5. Applying the Results of the Appraised Evidence:

Finally the evidence is integrated with clinical experience and patient values before applying it to the patient.

Ranking Quality of Evidence:

Systems to stratify evidence by quality have been developed for ranking evidence about the effectiveness of treatments or screening:

The U.S. Preventive Services Task Force System:

– <u>Level I:</u> Evidence obtained from at least one properly designed randomized controlled trial.

– <u>Level II-1:</u> Evidence obtained from well-designed controlled trials without randomization.

– <u>Level II-2:</u> Evidence obtained from well-designed cohort or case-control analytic studies, preferably from more than one center or research group.

– <u>Level II-3:</u> Evidence obtained from multiple time series with or without the intervention. Dramatic results in uncontrolled trials might also be regarded as this type of evidence.

– <u>Level III:</u> Opinions of respected authorities, based on clinical experience, descriptive studies, or reports of expert committees.

The RCOG System:

– <u>Level Ia:</u> Evidence obtained from meta-analysis of randomized controlled trials.

– <u>Level Ib:</u> Evidence obtained from at least one randomized controlled trial.

– <u>Level IIa:</u> Evidence obtained from at least one well-designed controlled study without randomization.

- Level IIb: Evidence obtained from at least one other type of well-designed quasi-experimental study.
- Level III: Evidence obtained from well-designed non-experimental descriptive studies, such as comparative studies, correlation studies and case studies.
- Level IV: Evidence obtained from expert committee reports or opinions and/or clinical experience of respected authorities.

Grades of Recommendations:

In guidelines and other publications, recommendation for a clinical service is classified by:
- The balance of risk versus benefit of the service, and
- The level of evidence on which this information is based.

The U.S. Preventive Services Task Force System:

- Level A: Good scientific evidence suggests that the benefits of the clinical service substantially outweigh the potential risks. Clinicians should discuss the service with eligible patients.
- Level B: At least fair scientific evidence suggests that the benefits of the clinical service outweigh the potential risks. Clinicians should discuss the service with eligible patients.
- Level C: At least fair scientific evidence suggests that there are benefits provided by the clinical service, but the balance between benefits and risks are too close for making general recommendations. Clinicians need not offer it unless there are individual considerations.

– Level D: At least fair scientific evidence suggests that the risks of the clinical service outweigh potential benefits. Clinicians should not routinely offer the service to patients.

– Level I: Scientific evidence is lacking, of poor quality, or conflicting, such that the risk versus benefit balance cannot be assessed. Clinicians should help patients understand the uncertainty surrounding the clinical service.

The RCOG System:

– Level A: Requires at least one randomized controlled trial as part of a body of literature of overall good quality and consistency addressing the specific recommendation.

– Level B: Requires the availability of well controlled clinical studies but no randomized clinical trials on the topic of recommendations.

– Level C: Requires evidence obtained from expert committee reports or opinions and/or clinical experiences of respected authorities; indicates an absence of directly applicable clinical studies of good quality.

2- *Setting*

Setting of the study gives a scientific power because the study done in a qualified institute will definitely be better than that done in a non-qualified place.

Research standards and supervision will definitely be powerful in the former.

Brief description of the study place convinces the reader in its importance.

Avoid vague titles "an academic medical center" or "a big medical institute" because this will generate a doubt in the reader's mind.

Duration of the study should be mentioned and should be suitable to the size of the study; e.g. the study was performed during the period from ... to...

Sample characteristics are also an important thing to mention; you should report your sample type (either random or non-random sample) as well as sample size and if you calculated that sample size or simple chosen on fund or equipment base.

Sample size calculation must be done in all studies aimed to be powerful enough to change traditional practice or thinking.

3- *Participants*

You must have clear description of your study participants (previously known as patients, subjects or cases):

Inclusion Criteria:

- Clear definition of the included participants' characteristics.
- Clear definition of the included pathology.
- Clear definition of the presentation.

Exclusion Criteria:

All individuals with any confounding characteristics should be excluded from the study participants.

Confounders are non-study variables that may affect the outcomes of the study; e.g. diabetes is a confounder when you study treatment of moniliasis because diabetic cases are more resistant to monilia treatment than non-diabetic cases.

Control Group:

Contrary to what is usually believed, the size of the control group should be at least equal to that of the cases groups and better to be larger.

Controls are sometimes problematic because there may be no way to recruit them simple in the study; this will take much effort to search for such suitable individuals without biasing the study.

You should explain clearly the size, characteristics and sources of the control group especially if the controls are normal healthy individuals.

Group Assignment in Clinical Trials:

In all clinical trials, you should describe how did you allocated the study participants into groups.

It is well known that randomized trials are much more powerful than non-randomized ones.

If you performed a randomized trial, you should describe:
− The method of randomization used (coin toss, dice rolling, sealed envelopes or random number table),
− Who did randomization, and
− How this randomization is concealed.

Example: The study population was randomly assigned to either treatment or placebo group. The randomization process was performed using a computer-generated random number table. Assignments were sealed in identical opaque envelops saved with the library secretary and were opened after enrollment.

Long Scenario:

Many of the journals now request a flow chart to show the participants track line throughout the study.

The following chart shows the scenario of enrolling the participants in the study:

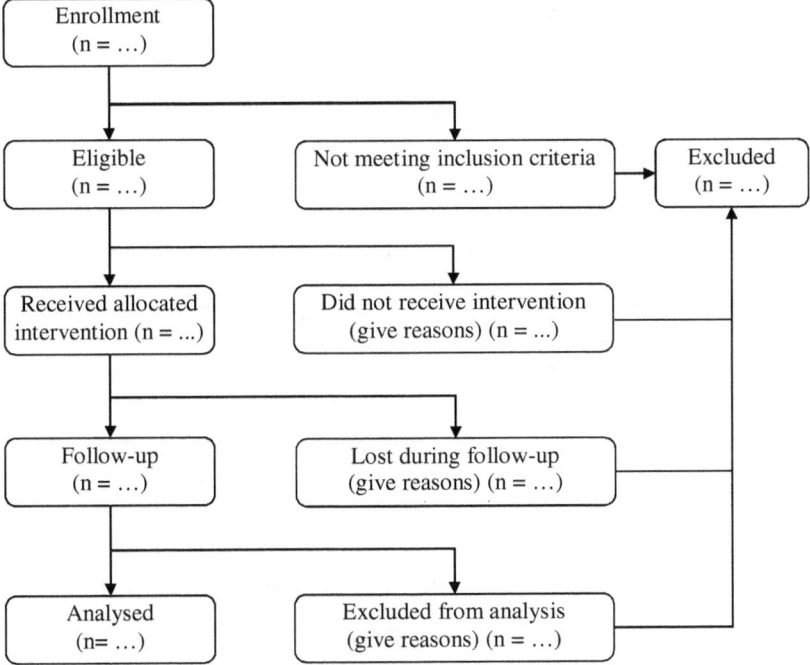

Flow Chart

4- *Interventions*

This part starts usually by reporting the human rights committee approval, ethical committee approval, consent or explanation; this may be the first part written in the subjects and methods.

Important basic signs and special investigations are first described briefly to include or exclude cases and as preliminary to study investigations.

Study investigation starts in a new paragraph:
- Enough details of tools, machines, instruments and kits (trade name, model, source and contact data).
- Specify critical values.
- Specify effect size needed to be found.
- Old techniques are briefly described with references.
- Modifications of standard techniques are fully described with methodology references.

If you did something unusual or used an unfamiliar method, you must explain.

If you are giving placebo in a clinical trial, you must describe how the study drug cannot be differentiated from placebo.

5- *Follow-up*

For how long?

– Your follow-up must be enough to cover all study outcomes.

What was done?

– Follow-up investigations should be complete and efficient to evaluate all possible outcomes.

What interval?

– The interval of the follow-up should be adjusted to record all possible changes in the course of all the studied outcomes.

Blinding:

Blindness is ensuring that a person remains unaware of the type of intervention a subject has been allocated to until the end of the study.

If possible, both the patients and the observers should be blinded to the given treatment; this makes better results especially if the outcome is opinion based.

It is important to decrease tendency to report more favorable outcomes in the control group, and less favorable outcomes in the control group; and to decrease bias in measuring outcome by investigators (ascertainment bias).

Trials are often described as:

- Single blinded: Blinding the subjects participating in the trial.
- Double blinded: Blinding the subjects and investigators (clinicians, interviewers, laboratory personnel).
- Triple blinded: Blinding the subjects, investigators and committee responsible for monitoring outcome as well as persons who perform data entry, analysis and statistics.

Important types of bias in RCTs:

- Selection bias: Improper patient selection and allocation to treatment groups.
- Ascertainment bias: Bias in recording and analyzing data.
- Dropout bias: Mishandling of patients who drop-out the study.
- Publication bias: Publishing only trials with positive and ignoring those with negative results.

Dropouts:

The longer the follow up, the higher the dropout participants; it is logic to think that dropouts will affect the validity and power of the study.

Although there is no universally accepted cutoff, a dropout of 20% of participants will considerably affect the study.

So, you should, as much as possible, report how many the dropouts in your study and why they are dropped out.

It is a common practice to exclude dropouts as they represent missing data and analyze the rest of participants (called "per-protocol analysis").

This may be accepted in descriptive or observational studies (although still will affect the validity and power); yet it is never accepted in clinical trials because it may lead to overestimation of the treatment effect which is very dangerous in such type of research.

Intension to Treat Analysis:

This means that all participants will be analyzed as they were randomized whether completed the study or dropped out.

Advantages of intension to treat analysis:
− Preserves randomization.
− Bias in the conservative direction.

Disadvantages of intension to treat analysis:
May lead to underestimation of the treatment effect, however, this is safer for the patient.

Worst Case Scenario:

All dropouts from the study group will be considered bad outcomes, and all dropouts from the control group will be considered good outcome.

6- *Outcome Measures*

Every researcher should clearly state the outcomes of the research; outcomes may be:

1- Primary Outcome(s):

These are the principal outcome(s) of the research; e.g. example: treatment of anovulation; treatment of osteoporosis.

The researcher should always choose patient oriented outcomes rather than disease oriented outcomes; e.g. in a research about treatment of anovulation, pregnancy is a patient oriented outcome while ovulation is a disease oriented outcome; in a research about treating osteoporosis, frequency of fractures is a patient oriented outcome while bone mineral density is a disease oriented outcome.

2- Secondary Outcome(s):

These are other outcomes than the principal one(s); e.g. the primary outcome in a research may be success of certain treatment for certain disease.

However, the research also studies side effects and complications, patient compliance, cost, etc. as secondary outcomes.

7- *Statistical Analysis*

We are not obliged to perform statistical analysis of our researches, or to understand the theory underlying the procedures.

Yet, we have to know enough to write about the rationale for using the tests, or at least to edit what your statistical colleagues have written.

Essential statistics:
— Methods of data description.
— Methods of data analysis.
— Data distribution.
— Data transformation.
— Adjustment of results.
— Critical P values for statistical significance.
— The used program (name, version, source).

Introduction to Biomedical Statistics:

Scientific research follows a "4-steps approach" known as the scientific method:

1. Observation,

2. Hypothesis,

3. Experiment, and

4. Conclusion.

1. Observation:

Research always starts by an observation.

2. Hypothesis:

The observation is used to formulate a research question using the "Null Hypothesis".

"There is no association between 2 variables" or

"There is no association between 2 groups":

– Exposure and harm.

– Preventive strategy and spread of a disease.

– Intervention and cure from a disease.

Example:

Observation: Cancer breast is more common in postmenopausal women on HRT.

Question: Does HRT use increase the incidence of cancer breast in postmenopausal women?

Null hypothesis: "There is no difference in the incidence of cancer breast in postmenopausal women on HRT and those who are not on HRT."

3. The Study:

The study design plays a crucial role for the validity of the study; each research question has a specific study design to answer:

– Therapy --- RCT.

– Harm and etiology --- Cohort and case-control studies.

4. Drawing Conclusions:

Why to use statistics?

We try to make use of the certainties of mathematics to solve the uncertainties of biology.

Can we draw conclusions from a sample and apply it to the whole population?

This is what statistics try to answer:

- If the difference between the outcomes did not occur by chance (P value is <0.05), we can reject the null hypothesis.

- If the difference between the outcomes has occurred by chance (P value is ≥0.05), we can accept the null hypothesis.

Statistics:

- The science concerned with data management.
- The science of measuring uncertainty.
- The science of measuring the known sources of variation.
- The art of drawing correct conclusions from inaccurate data.

Data management includes:

- Organization, summarization and description of data (descriptive statistics).
- Analysis of data to draw statistical conclusions and make statistical decisions (analytical statistics).

Descriptive Statistics:

Statistical methods that summarize a large set of data into a few meaningful numbers.

Data are broadly classified into:

- Numerical (quantitative) data.
- Categorical (qualitative) data.

Numerical (Quantitative) Data:

Data that are basically represented in numbers such as age, weight, height, temperature, blood pressure, etc…

Characteristics of Quantitative Data:
− Numerically represented.
− Accurate representation of data.
− All mathematical rules can be correctly applied.
− Analyzed by the most powerful statistical methods.

Distribution of Data:

To draw the mostly correct conclusions by statistics, you must determine how frequent each value had occurred in the studied data; this is called data distribution.

Determination of data distribution is an important requirement to do correct statistics.

When a graph is drawn to show the frequency of occurrence of each value in a data set, this is called data distribution graph (histogram).

If most of data are in the middle range and the extreme values are equally rare, the shape of the curve will be symmetrically bell shaped; this is called the "normal distribution", otherwise it is called "non-normal distribution".

Normal

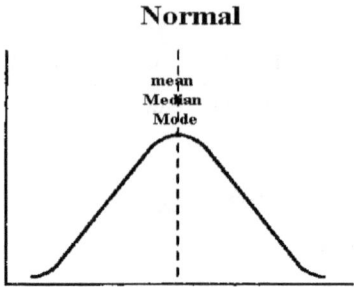

Rt Tailed (Skewed Rt or +ve skew)

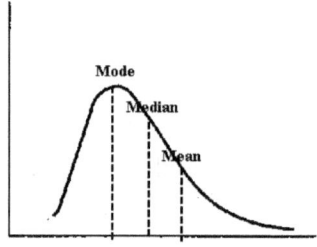

Lt Tailed (Skewed Lt or -ve skew)

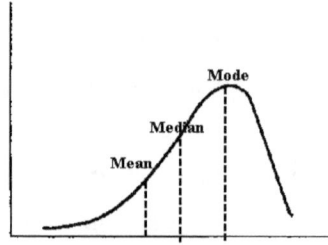

Data Distribution

Normally distributed data are analyzed using what is known as "parametric tests", while non-normal data are analyzed using "non-parametric tests".

Parametric statistics is generally more powerful than non-parametric statistics in making decisions and conclusions and should always be used whenever possible.

Non-normal data can be made normal by what is known as "data transformation". The most famous method of transformation is calculating the log values.

Description of Numerical Data:
− Measures of central tendency (location)

Mean

Median

Mode

− Measures of variation (dispersion)

Range

Standard deviation

− Frequency distribution

I- Measures of central tendency (location):

These are values that represent the middle or midpoint of the possible values of a variable.

The most famous measures of central tendency are:

1- The Mean:

It is the arithmetic average of a set of numerical data.

It represents the central value of the data that depends on the size of the data values.

It is calculated by dividing the sum of the data values by the number of data.

Properties:
– There is only one mean for each set of data.
– It is affected by every single value in the data set (any change in any single value will change the mean); so it is a sensitive measure.
– It is not necessary to be equal to any of the data values.

It is most suitable for normally distributed quantitative data especially of large number of records.

In data with few records or many extreme values (outliers) the use of arithmetic mean is of low value.

2- The Median:

It is the middle value of a ranked array (it divides the array into 2 equal parts).

If the total number of series values is even, the median is the arithmetic mean of the 2 middle values.

Properties:
— Only one median is present for each data set.
— It represents the position rather than the amount of the values in the data set.
— It is not affected by the other values in the data array. So it is less sensitive than the mean.
— It is not necessary to be equal to any of the data values.

It is of special importance in non-normal quantitative data, and data with many outliers.

3- The Mode:

It is the most frequently occurring value.

Some series have no mode while others have more than one mode.

It must be equal to one or more value in the data set.

II- Measures of Variation (Dispersion):

Describe the data variations around the central measure.

1- The Range:

Most suitable with the median.

It is the difference between the maximum and minimum values in the data set.

Sometimes the range may be calculated between 2 reference values not the maximum and the minimum.

When the range is between the 1st and 3rd quarters of the data it is called the interquartile range.

Properties:
− Easy measure of the dispersion.
− It is not representative of all data.
− It is affected only by the maximum and minimum values. So it may be misleading when there is a single extreme value in the data set (outliers).

2- The Variance and Standard Deviation:

Variance is the mean of squared deviation around the mean.

It represents an index of the spread of measurements around the mean.

It describes subject-to-subject variation within the data array.

It is more sensitive than the range because it is affected by every value in the data set.

It is not practical because the deviation is squared, so to be practical, its value should be square rooted which gives the **standard deviation (SD)** which is most suitable with the arithmetic mean.

A range of one SD above and below the mean (abbreviated to ± 1 SD) includes 68.2% of the values.

± 2 SD includes 95.4% of the data.

± 3 SD includes 99.7%.

Coefficient of Variation:

It is the parentage of SD: mean ratio (SD ÷ mean × 100).

It has the advantages of nullifying the effect of the unit of measurement of the variable. So, it is useful to compare 2 sets of data with different units of measurements (temperature measured in Celsius and Kelvin) and in cases when data have equal SD but different arithmetic means.

III- Frequency Distribution:

If we transformed numerical data into categories, it is possible to describe through frequency tables.

Each row in the table represents a "class" and the range of the class is called the "class interval"; ideally, the class interval should be equal.

Categorical (Qualitative) Data:

Data not represented basically in numbers such as sex, race, blood groups, hair color, etc…

Characteristics of Qualitative Data:

– Less accurate representation of data (depends on estimation rather than measure).
– Mathematical rules cannot be correctly applied.
– Analyzed by less powerful statistical methods.

Qualitative data are classified into:

1- Nominal Data:

Data which can be categorized but with no specific order (not ranked) e.g. sex, color of hair, race, religion, blood groups, etc…

Dichotomous data are type of nominal data the result of which may be one of 2 responses e.g. occurrence of pregnancy, menopausal status, etc. and are also called Bernoulli or binary data.

Polychotomous data are those with more than 2 responses e.g. blood group A, B, AB, or O; white, black, yellow, oriental race, etc...

2- Ordinal Data:

Ordered (ranked) data e.g. severity scale (mild, moderate, severe); tumor stages, scoring systems, etc.

Description of Categorical Data:

Categorical Data can be described as:
− Number
− Fraction
− Percent

Frequency is the number of times of the occurrence of an event.

Relative frequency is the number of times of the occurrence of an event as a fraction (or percent) of the total.

Cumulative frequency is the fraction (or percentage) of observations that are less than the upper limit of each interval.

Frequency measures are the only way to describe categorical data and are used to describe numerical data when transformed into categories.

The 2×2 frequency table formed of only 2 columns and 2 rows (the totals are not counted).

Statistical Inference and Confidence Interval (CI):

So long as samples are subsets of populations, thus calculations on samples can be used as estimates (called statistics) of those of the population (called parameters).

Thus, the mean of a sample is considered an estimate for the mean of the population from which the sample is withdrawn; and the sample variance is considered as an estimate for population variance, and so on.

However, despite proper sampling method, there is always a probability of difference between the sample "statistic" and the true population "parameter" as well as a difference between any sample and the other.

This is because no sample can represent the population 100% as most of the population individuals are not included in any sample whatever is.

So, it is logic to expect that any statistic will differ (slightly) from the true population parameter as well as from sample to sample (whatever perfect is it).

Thus it is not possible to know the true population parameters from any sample.

This will make no sample is trustful to reflect the population values.

Although we cannot know the true population parameters using any sample, it is possible to calculate a range or an interval in which we will be confident that the true population parameters lie inside.

This concept is called "statistical inference" and the interval is called the "confidence interval (CI)".

This interval can be calculated from one single done sample.

Calculation of the CI depends on calculating the amount of change of the estimate from sample to sample, this is called the standard error (SE) and this, in turn, depends on the amount of variation in the sample and the sample size.

Thus, the higher the variation in the done sample (e.g. SD) the higher the SE and the smaller the sample size, the higher the SE and vice versa.

A last point; this CI is actually estimated, how much can I trust this interval in including the true population parameter?

There is a general agreement that 95% confidence is enough and a 5% error will not affect the statistical results.

Analytical Statistics:

The aim of statistical analysis is to investigate the differences or to make relation between different sets of data.

This is useful to make statistical conclusions and decisions; statistical conclusions and decisions help clinical decisions *but do not determinate clinical decisions*.

Aspects of Statistical Analysis:
1- Statistical comparison.
2- Correlation and regression.
3- Sensitivity and specificity.

Statistical Comparison:

Statistical comparisons aim to detect if sample difference is significant (associated with population difference) or non-significant (not associated with population difference and is due to chance).

The answer lies in the p value that will result from the statistical test whatever is.

This p value is the probability of chance.

The *P* (Probability) Value:

There is a general agreement that if the probability of chance is <0.05 (*P* value <5%) we can safely conclude that the difference is real and not due to chance, while if the *P* value is 0.05 or more, we can conclude that the difference is due to chance.

We can also formulate the original question in another way; we can assume that there is no difference between the groups and then ask whether this assumption is right or wrong.

The assumption of "no difference" is called the "null hypothesis" (the hypothesis of no difference, H_0) and we ask whether the H_0 is true or false.

If the *P* value is <0.05, this means that the probability of chance is low, thus the difference is significant, thus we can reject the null hypothesis and H_0 is false.

If the *P* value is ≥0.05, this means that the probability of chance is considerable, thus the difference is non-significant, thus we accept the null hypothesis and H_0 is true.

The lower the *P* value, the less likely it is that the difference happened by chance and so the higher the significance of the finding.

$P = 0.01$ is often considered to be "highly significant"; it means that the difference will only have happened by chance 1 in 100 times, this is unlikely, but still possible.

$P = 0.001$ means the difference will have happened by chance 1 in 1000 times, even less likely, but still just possible; it is usually considered to be "very highly significant".

Which test I choose?

Student's *t* Test:

This test is typically used to compare just two samples of "normally distributed" data.

Mann-Whitney *U* Test:

This test is used to compare two samples when the data are not normally distributed.

Analysis of Variance (ANOVA):

This is a group of statistical techniques used to compare two or more samples of "normally distributed" data.

Kruskal Wallis Test:

This test is used to compare two or more samples when the data are not normally distributed.

Chi-square (χ^2) Test:

It is a measure of the difference between actual and expected frequencies.

The "expected frequency" is that there is no difference between the sets of results (the null hypothesis); in that case, the χ^2 value would be zero.

The larger the actual difference between the sets of results, the greater the χ^2 value.

However, it is difficult to interpret the χ^2 value by itself as it depends on the number of factors studied; statisticians make it easier by giving the p value.

Fisher's Exact Test:

Instead of the χ^2 test, "Fisher's exact test" is sometimes used to analyze contingency tables as it always gives the exact p value, particularly where the numbers are small.

The following chart shows the basic concept of choosing comparison tests:

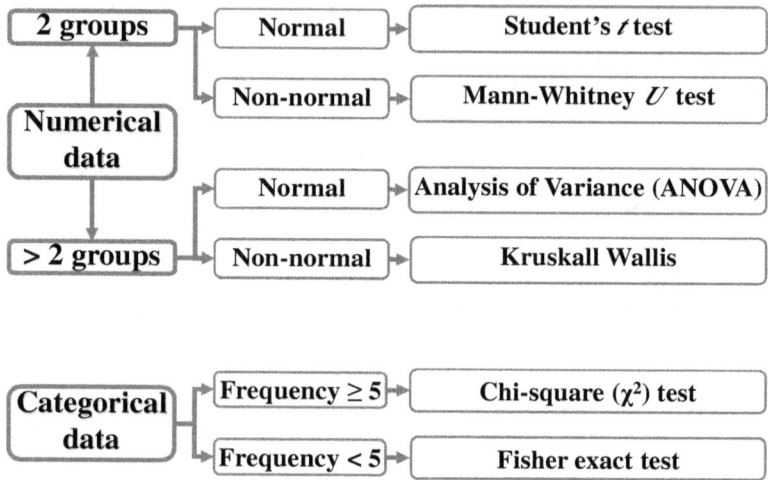

Statistical Comparison

Correlation and Regression:

Sometimes you notice that in two series of quantitative or ordinal data, the values of one variable may vary correspondingly with the other one.

For example, it is well known that as age increases in children, the height increases as well, also, in old age as age increases the bone mineral density decreases as well; this relation is called "correlation".

When the two variables increase and decrease in parallel (same direction), this called "positive correlation".

If one variable goes and the other goes down proportionally (opposite directions), it is called "negative correlation".

Graphically, correlation is represented by what is known as the "scatter diagram".

In this diagram, each individual is represented by a dot that represents the values of the correlated variables; one variable is put on the X axis, and the other is put on the Y axis.

When the points on the scatter diagram represent a linear pattern, the correlation is termed "linear correlation" while if taking a curvilinear pattern it is "non-linear correlation".

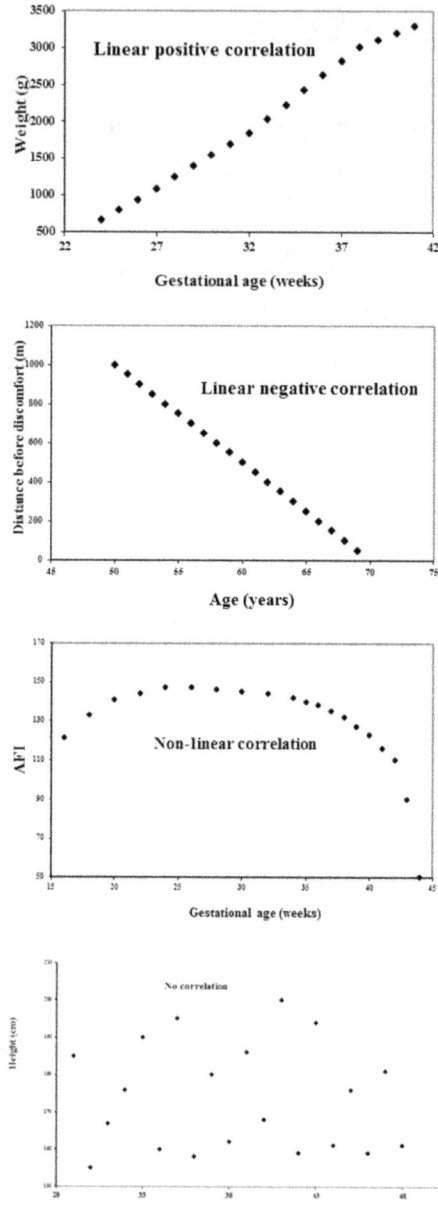

Correlation Studies

In normally distributed data, linear correlation is tested using the "Pearson's product moment correlation" method that depends on the calculation of the correlation coefficient "r".

The range of r is from 0 (means no correlation) to 1 (means perfect relation).

The "algebraic sign" means the direction of correlation and is not a value.

The following is a good rule of thumb when considering the size of a correlation:

$r = 0$–0.2: very low and probably meaningless.

$r = 0.2$–0.4: a low correlation that might warrant further investigation.

$r = 0.4$–0.6: a reasonable correlation.

$r = 0.6$–0.8: a high correlation.

$r = 0.8$–1.0: a very high correlation; check for errors or other reasons for such a high correlation.

This guide also applies to negative correlations.

In non-normally distributed data, correlation is tested using the "Spearman rank correlation" method which depends on calculating the correlation coefficient (ρ).

Regression:

Regression is a method used to derive an equation to estimate the value of one variable when the value of another correlated variable (or variables) is known.

If the equation includes two variables only, it is called "simple regression", while if there are more than two variables it is called "multivariable or multivariate or multiple regression". If one variable is binary, the regression model is called "logistic regression".

The graphic representation of regression is like correlation uses the scatter diagram with addition of a straight line representing the regression equation line; it is called the "trend line" or "regression line".

This line is passing on the maximum number of pints and is nearest to all points; thus every set of data will have a special trend line.

The regression coefficient gives the "slope" of the graph, in that it gives the change in value of one outcome, per unit change in the other.

This regression equation can be applied to any regression line; it is represented by: $y = a + b x$

To predict the value "y" (value on the vertical axis of the graph) from the value "x" (on the horizontal axis), "b" is the regression coefficient and "a" is the constant.

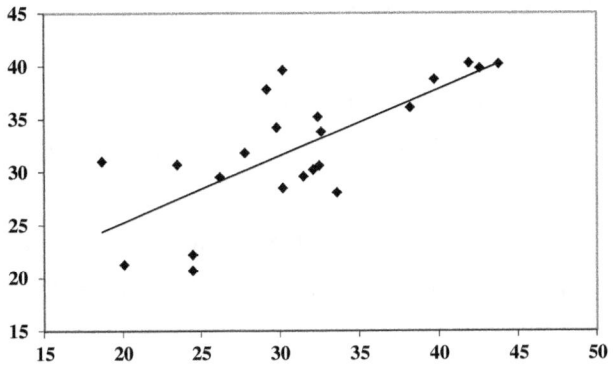

Trend "Regression" Line

Correlation and regression are generally needed when there is one variable difficult to measure and another one easy to measure.

If both variables are correlated, we can use the easy measured variable to estimate the value of the difficult to measure variable.

Correlation measures the *strength* of the association between variables.

Regression *quantifies* the association; it should only be used if one of the variables is thought to precede or cause the other.

Sensitivity and Specificity:

To calculate the accuracy of the new diagnostic test, a sample of individuals is exposed to both the new test and a suitable gold standard.

According to the results of the gold standard, the participants are divided into diseased and non-diseased while according to the results of the new diagnostic test, the participants are divided into test positive and negative.

True +ve:
Are cases diagnosed +ve by the new test and proved to be diseased by the gold standard.

True -ve:
Are cases diagnosed -ve by the new test and proved to be non-diseased by the gold standard.

False +ve:
Are cases diagnosed +ve by the new test but proved to be non-diseased by the gold standard.

False -ve:
Are cases diagnosed -ve by the new test but proved to be diseased by the gold standard.

How Accurate is the Test?

Sensitivity:

It is the proportion of diseased individuals who are diagnosed +ve by the new test (true +ve).

Sensitivity = true +ve / all diseased cases in the study (which is true +ve + false -ve).

Specificity:

It is the proportion of non-diseased subjects who are diagnosed -ve by the new test (true -ve).

Specificity = True -ve / all non-diseased cases in the study (which is true -ve + False +ve).

Overall accuracy:

It is the proportion of those who were truly diagnosed in the study to the total number.

Overall accuracy = (True +ve + true -ve) / (all subjects).

Does the Patient Have the Disease or Not?

Although sensitivity and specificity have been used for a long time to evaluate the accuracy of new diagnostic tests, yet they are not useful to evaluate the usefulness of the test in helping a particular patient.

Suppose that the patient has a positive (or a negative) test, the question to be answered is not how much accurate is the test but the question that the patient needs an answer to is "given this test result; what is my probability of having the disease?"

These indices are known as the predictive values:

Positive Predictive Value (PPV):

It is the probability of a patient with a positive test to have the disease.

PPV = true +ve / all +ve.

Negative Predictive Value (NPV):

It is the probability of a patient with a negative test to be free of the disease.

NPV = true -ve / all -ve.

Unfortunately the predictive values of a test are not constant as they depend on the prevalence of the disease in the population, i.e. they change with the increase or the decrease of the prevalence.

In other words they change with the pre-test probability of the disease as prevalence is considered the probability of having the disease.

The Likelihood Ratio:

From the above it is clear that what is important in helping a particular patient is how much the test is able to change our minds from what we thought before the test (pre-test probability) to what we think afterward (post-test probability).

The diagnostic tests that produce big changes from pretest to post-test probabilities are the important tests and likely to be useful to us in our practice.

The new practical way to express the usefulness of a diagnostic test is calculating the likelihood ratios of positive test (LR +ve) and of negative test (LR -ve).

The Likelihood Ratio of a Positive Test (LR +ve):

LR +ve = Sensitivity / (100 - specificity).

The more is the LR +ve the better is the test to increase the probability of the presence of the disorder.

LR +ve = 1 means no use of the test (no change between the pretest probability and posttest probability).

The Likelihood Ratio of a Negative Test (LR -ve):

LR -ve = (100 - sensitivity) / Specificity.

The less is the LR -ve the better is the test to decrease the probability of presence of the disorder.

LR -ve = 1 means no use of the test (no change between the pretest probability and posttest probability).

The likelihood ratios are used with the pretest probability to determine the posttest probability.

Key Message:

"Statistical thinking will one day be as necessary a qualification for efficient citizenship as the ability to read and write." *Wells H.G.*

V- Results

It is the core "heart" of the paper; it gives the facts, summarizes and visualizes them for the reader, but excludes any discussion.

You should present only relevant and representative data without duplication.

Use well designed tables to summarize details and illustrative figures to give impressions.

Presentation of Data:

1- Text:
Start with some text then refer the reader to a table or figure where they can see the data for themselves.

2- Tables:
Best suited to direct attention to individual pieces of numeric information and statistical validity.

3- Figures:
– Charts or graphs: Used to show trends and emphasize comparisons between the important points.
– Pictures: e.g. X-ray, US, pathology …

Common chart types:

- Bar chart: Shows discrete values using columns.

- Line chart: Shows values as connected points by lines to show trends and comparisons.

- Pie chart: Shows how individual data values contribute to an overall total (percentages).

- Scatter plot: Plots two sets of potentially related data to identify possible association.

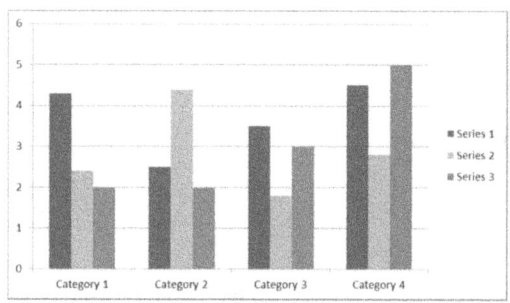

Bar Chart

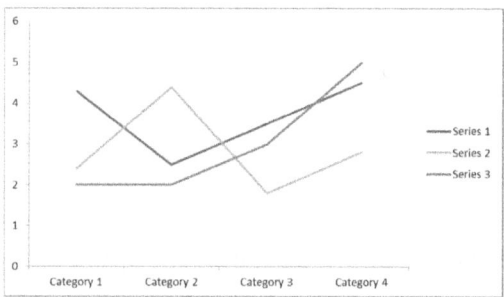

Line Chart

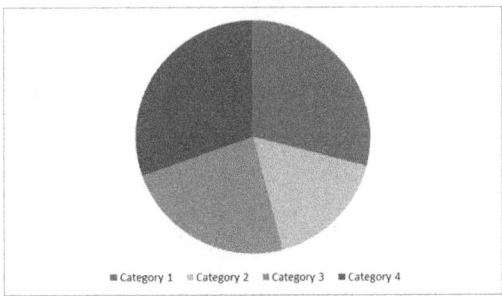

Pie Chart

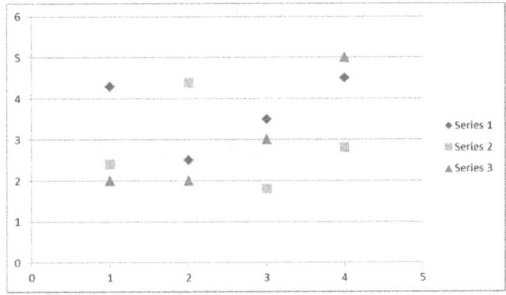

Scatter Plot

VI- <u>DISCUSSION</u>

This section tells us what your results mean, why they are important and how they fit in with existing knowledge.

It is the place where you state the answer of your research question, supported by your main results and existing knowledge about the topic.

The discussion is also where you point out alternative explanations for your findings and argue why you think your interpretation is the best (or tell us what further test is needed to show which hypothesis is correct).

It is an exercise in logic and discipline; it should be focused, and can be structured.

Be clear and specific about the interpretation of your results and the implications of your work.

You should summarize your main findings, compare your work with others and justify any differences.

You should also acknowledge errors (and convince us why they do not alter your conclusion).

Strengths and limitations of the study should be mentioned as well as clinical implications discussed, and future thoughts initiated, ending up by a very specific conclusion.

The Main Components of Discussion:

– Answer to the research question.

– Support for the answer (main results).

– Explanation for the answer.

– Argument with and against other research findings.

– Unexpected and surprising results (if any).

– Limitations of the study.

– Importance and newness of work.

Answer the Research Question:

– The most important part of the discussion, so keep it the first part.

– Signal the answer, e.g.: Our study shows ...

– Use the same key terms as the question.

– Use the present tense.

– Include the population to whom the answer generalizes.

Support the Answer:

– Support your answer with the most relevant results.

– For signaling, e.g.: The evidence is that ...

– Do not expect the reader has memorized all your results.

– Cite appropriate tables or figures when needed.

Explain the Answer:

– Why it is reasonable?

– What is the biological basis for your answer?

Defend the Answer:

− How does it fit with previously published reports?

− If there is other possible answers for your question.

− Argue for your answer.

− Argue against the other answers.

Unexpected and Surprising Results:

− Results that do not support your hypothesis or are surprising.

− Mention them in separate paragraph; in the beginning of the paragraph you must mention that they were unexpected findings, e.g.: Contrary to our hypothesis, we were surprised that...

− Try to explain them.

Study Limitations:

− If your study has limitations (and everyone has) you must mention them.

− Limitations could be related to design or methods.

− Readers and editors are most interested in your study limitations

Importance of Work:

− At the end of discussion.

− Mention what you added to the already known about the subject.

− Mention applications, recommendations, implications or speculations.

− Avoid claiming priority, e.g.: this is the first ever report about..!

− If you are very sure say: To the best of our knowledge this is the first report describing ...

Organization of the Discussion:

The Beginning:

- Answer the question:

  Only state the answer.

  Start with the study question followed by the answer.

  Provide a brief context then state the answer.

- Support the answer

The Middle:

- Explain and defend the answer within the context of existing knowledge.
- Divide the body of your discussion into subsections and each subsection into paragraphs.
- Start each subsection by a topic sentence that indicates the message of the section.
- Mention conflicting results, unexpected events and try to explain them.

The End:

- The conclusion is the end of discussion
- For signaling the conclusion, e.g.: In conclusion; To summarize.
- Usually it includes restatement of the answer to the study question.
- It also includes the importance of the findings with their potential implications.
- Any suggestions for further studies or future research

VII- **References**

References are your sources of information; you should state the source of any ideas, facts, tables, figures, quotations, research, techniques, etc. in your article.

Citations allow the reader to follow up those ideas and facts, to check your interpretation of that information and to replicate your work in other settings.

References in a manuscript are needed in three main areas:
- Introduction (Background References),
- Methods (Methodological references), and
- Discussion (References for relevant studies).

Background References:

They are needed to affirm the importance of the topic, to demonstrate your familiarity with existing knowledge in the field, to emphasize the presence of gap in the literature and to justify your research question.

Choose only a few (5-10), a recent review of the literature may be preferable to citing 10 or 20 original articles; however, groundbreaking articles should be cited and an extensive reference list cannot substitute for a thorough review of the literature.

You should read every reference; and demonstrate that you understood the implications of each study.

Take care that references to review articles can be an efficient way of guiding readers to a body of literature; however, review articles do not always reflect original work accurately.

Readers should therefore be provided with direct references to original research sources whenever possible.

Methodological References:

They provide other investigators with sources of your methods; verify the validity of your results and allow replication of your work by other researchers.

Cite the original reference for any measurement using an assay, instrument, or questionnaire that has been used previously, and then explain in a sentence or two.

Provide enough detail if you are the first to describe the technique, if you present a modification of an already known measurement or if reference is obscure.

Provide references for classification of disease, diagnostic criteria of disease, critical values used and sources and addresses of kits and equipment.

References in Discussion Section:

They are needed to compare your work with others and justify your findings.

Include about 10 to 20 references of focused, up to date, prior studies that agree or disagree with your results, provide a biological explanation for your results, suggest clinical relevance or indicate that a similar phenomenon has been observed in other settings

Common References Styles:

− Name-and-Year-System (Harvard) e.g. El-Mazny et al., 2011.
− Citation-Sequence-System (the numerical or Vancouver system), e.g. (1, 2, 4); required in the Uniform Requirements of International Committee of Medical Journal Editors "ICMJE".

The Uniform Requirements style is based largely on a standard style adapted by the National Library of Medicine (NLM) for its databases.

The essential details required are (in order):

Journal articles:

− Name/s of author/s, editor/s, compiler/s or the institution responsible. Where there are 7 or more authors, only the first 6 are listed and add "et al" (means "and others").
− Title of article and subtitle if any.
− Title of journal (abbreviated according to the style used in Index Medicus).

– Year (and month/day if necessary/available) of publication.

– Volume number (and issue/part).

– Page ranges.

Example:

El-Mazny A, Abou-Salem N. A double-blind randomized controlled trial of vaginal misoprostol for cervical priming before outpatient hysteroscopy. Fertil Steril. 2011 Oct; 96 (4): 962-5.

Book references:

– Name/s of author/s, editor/s, compiler/s or the institution responsible. Where there are 7 or more authors, only the first 6 are listed and add "et al".

– Title of publication and subtitle if any.

– Edition, if other than first edition.

– Publisher, the publisher's name should be spelt out in full.

– Year of publication.

Example:

El-Mazny A. Polycystic Ovary Syndrome: Pathogenesis and Management. LAMBERT Academic Publishing; 2011.

Basic Rules:

− Do not use a long list (20 to 40 are sufficient), use only those in indexed peer-reviewed journals.

− Never use a reference that you have not read.

− Never repeat a statement with its reference without verification.

− Do not rely solely on reading the abstract of a paper as it may be misleading or inaccurate.

− It is quite common for articles to be misinterpreted and/or misquoted with mistakes being perpetuated for many years by subsequent authors.

− Statements of fact must be referenced (except if so obvious).

− The results section should almost never have any reference citations; these may belong in the methods or discussion section.

− References cited only in tables or figure legends, should be numbered in accordance with the sequence established by the first identification in the text of the particular table or figure.

− Citations should be in numerical order.

− References should be numbered consecutively, in the order they are first mentioned in the text.

− Follow the journal's rules about how citations should appear in the text. Some journals prefer that citations be placed in parentheses; others ask for brackets; others want a superscript.

− Use dashes if there are several consecutive references (1-5, not 1, 2, 3, 4, 5).

− Attach references to the appropriate phrase within a sentence so that they are clearly linked, (Some studies [1-3] mentioned ..., contrary to others [4-6] who found that ...), otherwise, cite references for a particular sentence in chronological order, oldest to most recent.

- A single citation or string of citations, at the end of a paragraph, is not accepted.
- Avoid using abstracts as references, or at least, use them within 2 years.
- References to papers accepted but not yet published should be designated as "in press" or "forthcoming".
- Information from manuscripts submitted but not accepted should be cited in the text as "unpublished observations" with written permission from the source.
- Avoid citing a "personal communication" unless it provides essential information not available from a public source, in such case, the name of the person and date of communication should be cited in parentheses in the text. Authors should obtain written permission and confirmation of accuracy from the source of a personal communication.
- Avoid citation errors; typographical and spelling errors are common in reference lists, some journals check the accuracy of all reference citations, but not all journals. To minimize such errors, authors should therefore verify references against the original documents. Always redo your literature search and references, and up-date them each time you submit, or re-submit, a manuscript.

Chapter III:

Research Publishing

"Publish or perish" is an old saying that is very true, now more than ever.

"It is not an easy task but gives great joy" despite all the obstacles we face.

Research work is incomplete unless the results are disseminated to the wider community.

Publishing is important for yourself, your organization, your scientific colleagues and your funders.

It improves your career, since your work will be seen as good quality and reliable.

Why should you publish?
- To generalize knowledge,
- To improve patient care,
- To improves your writing and analytical skills,
- To achieve self-esteem,
- To have a place in international arena, and
- Ranking of Universities is related to the research output of the faculty, so "publish or your institute will perish".

Where should you publish?

Peer-reviewed journals are arguably the most widely respected avenue for presenting research findings.

Publishing in journals is also challenging – articles must follow strict guidelines and the rejection rate can be high.

Different journals cover different subject areas and regions.

Try to broaden your horizons; if you have just published in a national journal, aim for a regional or international journal.

Read journals – keep up to date and keep an eye open for where you think your work might fit in.

How to publish?

Publishing one's work is a challenge faced by every author, but it becomes easier with each new publication.

Most journals will provide "instructions for contributors" on how to publish in that journal.

This includes the layout and format of both the body and references of the article.

I- <u>UNIFORM REQUIREMENTS</u>

A small group of editors of general medical journals met informally in Vancouver, British Columbia, in 1978 to establish guidelines for the format of manuscripts submitted to their journals; this group became known as the "Vancouver Group".

Its requirements for manuscripts, including formats for bibliographic references developed by the National Library of Medicine, were first published in 1979.

The Vancouver Group expanded and evolved into the International Committee of Medical Journal Editors (ICMJE), which meets annually.

The ICMJE created the Uniform Requirements primarily to help authors and editors in their mutual task of creating and distributing accurate, clear, easily accessible reports of biomedical studies.

The initial sections address the ethical principles related to the process of evaluating, improving, and publishing manuscripts in biomedical journals and the relationships between editors and authors, peer reviewers, and the media.

The latter sections address the more technical aspects of preparing and submitting manuscripts.

Submission of an Article:

- Choose the appropriate journal according to its scope.
- Read "Instructions to the Author", adopt the Vancouver style, and follow the Uniform Requirements for Manuscripts Submitted to Biomedical Journals.
- Ensure that you have followed the journal's instructions including instructions for page layout, tables, figures and plates.
- Look at the printed copy, not the screen.
- Do not trust a spell checking program to find all the typographical errors.
- Look for errors in spelling, grammar, structure; consult an English language editor.
- Check the references.
- Make your submission polished.
- Submit electronically if possible.
- Write a polite covering letter in which you summarize why the work described in the manuscript is important and why you are submitting it to the journal – particularly important because the editor is not necessarily an expert in your field.
- Possibly recommend peer reviewers.
- Send the requested number of copies, number the pages, the tables and figures.
- Reviewers will regard a sloppy manuscript as evidence of sloppy work; your best chances for acceptance come with the editors' and reviewers' first impressions.

II- REVIEW PROCESS

Critical assessment of manuscripts submitted to journals should be performed by experts who are not part of the editorial staff; a process called peer review.

It helps editors decide which manuscripts are suitable for their journals, and helps authors and editors in their efforts to improve the quality of reporting.

A peer reviewed journal is one that submits most of its published research articles for outside review.

The number and kind of manuscripts sent for review, the number of reviewers, the reviewing procedures, and the use made of the reviewers' opinions may vary.

Each journal should publicly disclose its policies in its instructions to authors.

Reviewers Comment on:
− Scientific issues,
− Ethical issues, and
− The presentation of the manuscript.

Scientific Review Process:

- Is the work scientifically sound?
- Is the work an original contribution?
- Are the conclusions justified on the evidence presented?
- Are there any major errors in fact, logic or technique?
- Is the paper clearly and concisely written?
- Are the references appropriate, current and complete?

Ethical Review Process:

- Were the necessary ethical approvals obtained from a properly constituted and expert institutional ethics committee?
- Has the author declared any commercial, financial or other conflict of interest in the topic material?
- Has the author protected the patients' rights to privacy?

Review of the Presentation:

- Does the title clearly indicate the content of the paper?
- Does the abstract convey the essence of the article?
- Are the figures, diagrams and tables well-constructed and do they present the data effectively?
- Are all the illustrations, figures, diagrams and tables appropriate and essential for an understanding of the text?
- Are the illustrations and drawings of good quality and is the labeling adequate?
- Are the statistical methods appropriate and data properly presented?
- Are the references error-free and are they presented correctly?

Reviewers aim to exclude scientific fraud, plagiarism, and bias:

Scientific Fraud:

It is not the task of Editor to make full investigation or to make a determination.

It is the responsibility of the institution or funding agency, but the editor should be promptly informed.

If a fraudulent paper has been published, the journal must print a "retraction".

If the investigation did not result in a satisfactory conclusion, the editor may publish an "expression of concern" with an explanation.

Redundant or Duplicate Publication:

The publication of a paper overlaps with one already published, in print, or in electronic media conflicts with originality, and cost-effective use of resources.

If redundant publication is attempted, prompt rejection or notice if already published is presented to the authors.

Preliminary release to public media of scientific information described in a paper that has been accepted but not yet published, violates the policies of many journals.

Exceptions: Complete report following publication of a preliminary report or previous presentation at a scientific or professional meeting or press reports.

Precautions: This should be accompanied by a full statement to the editor about the situation; the published report should be referred to and referenced in the new paper, and copies of such material should be included with the submitted paper.

Outcome of Review:

– Rejection: Modify and submit to another journal.
– Rejection in the present form, reconsidered after major revision: Try to fix it or submit to another journal if you cannot change.
– Accept with modifications: Congratulations.
– Accept without modifications: Rare.

Possible comments:

Title:

– Shorten (5-15 words).
– Modify to reflect content.
– No abbreviations allowed.

Abstract:

− Stick to précised word count.

− Use structured format.

− Include all key data.

Introduction:

− Be concise and focused, quickly introduce the research question, and define the problem to be solved.

− Emphasize the gap of knowledge.

− Update some references, add important references.

− Appropriately use abbreviations.

Methods:

− Adequately describe (sampling, protocol, inclusion and exclusion criteria).

− Mention appropriate details of techniques.

− Precise the critical values used.

− Add important references.

− Emphasize the effect size.

Results:

− Present only relevant data.

− Do not duplicate, redesign or omit a table or figure.

− The text should complement the tables and figures.

− Clarify the effect size for the main outcome.

− Specify exact p values.

Discussion:

– Shorten the size.

– Omit the introduction.

– Focus on highly relevant studies.

– Justify the differences from other studies.

– Mention the limitations of the study.

– Suggest clinical implications.

– Reference pioneer work and major players.

– Should be very specific; don't generalize.

References:

– Update.

– Use Vancouver style.

– Stick to the format of the journal.

– Shorten the list.

– Add some important references.

Responding to Referee's Comments:

Respond to every comment, whether positive or negative, make changes only if you agree with them; if you do not change, you have to justify.

Address all comments – changes or otherwise – in a covering letter; remember the reviewer is not always right! Explain respectfully.

If there is no chance to win them over, provide a gentle statement for "unreasonable" criticisms that you are not addressing, you should still try and resolve some of their comments.

Things which must be done – change it, but things suggested that you think about – consider; consult others, who have the experience.

If the reviewer failed to understand, or overlooked already present data: probably the same will occur to the reader, make yourself more clear, concise and simple; point it out to him respectfully.

If the reviewer comments that you didn't reference some work (probably his own), he may get too hostile, try to add the reference.

Your attitude towards the reviewers' comments is important, all reviewers will read your statement of changes, and an accommodating approach is useful.

Other Changes in a Revised Manuscript:

Update the manuscript, if necessary, and correct mistakes from one version to the next; but always point such changes out.

A reviewer who notices changes that the authors did not acknowledge may write a hostile second review, including confidential comments to the editor.

Publication Bias:

Editors should consider seriously, for publication, any carefully done study of an important question, relevant to their readers, whether the results are negative or positive.

The Cochrane Library may be interested in publishing negative trials and insists on inclusion of unpublished studies in systematic reviews.

Conflicts of Interest:

All participants in the peer review and publication process must disclose all relationships that could be viewed as presenting a potential conflict of interest.

This is especially important in editorials and review articles, because it is can be more difficult to detect bias in these types of publications.

Editors should publish this information, if they believe it is important in judging the manuscript.

To prevent ambiguity, authors must state explicitly whether potential conflicts do or do not exist; authors should do so in the manuscript on a conflict of interest notification page that follows the title page, providing additional detail, if necessary, in a cover letter that accompanies the manuscript.

Editors' Tips:

– Study the journal; the first step is to know who the journal is for and the kinds of articles it publishes.

– Use good English; reviewers often reject papers because the grammar is bad, rather than on the basis of the content.

– Be realistic; be aware of the value of your results but don't over-interpret them.

– Tell a coherent story, and don't make sweeping conclusions if you don't have the results to support them; i.e. don't be over-speculative.

– Don't try too hard to sound important; don't use a pompous voice.

– Make sure the title matches the content

– Read lots of papers and learn from them.

Key Message:

– It is not an easy task but gives great joy.

– Learn time management, word processing, and research methodology and ethics.

– Be determined, gradual, gentle and realistic.

– Be perseverant and accommodating in journal submissions.

– Adopt what editors and reviewers want (excitement, importance of topic, originality, truth and clarity).

– There is always a hope to improve.

– "In science the credit goes to the man who convinces the world, not to the man to whom the idea first occurs." *Francis Darwin*

REFERENCES

- **Abalos E, Carroli G, Mackey M.** The tools and techniques of EBM. Best Pract Res Clin Obstet Gynaecol. 2005; 19: 15-26.
- **Albert T.** The A-Z of Medical Writing. London: BMJ Books; 2000.
- **Albert T.** Winning the publications game: How to write a scientific paper without neglecting your patients, 2nd ed. UK: Radcliffe Publishing Ltd; 2000.
- **Altman D.** Statistics in medical research. In: Practical statistics for medical research. London: Chapman and Hall; 1996.
- **Atkins D, Best D, Briss P.** Grading quality of evidence and strength of recommendations. BMJ. 2004; 328: 1490.
- **Bland M.** An introduction to medical statistics, 2nd ed. Oxford, UK: Oxford University Press; 1996.
- **Castle W, North P.** Statistics in Small Doses, 3rd ed. Edinburgh, UK: Churchill Livingstone; 1995.
- **Eddy D.** Evidence-based medicine: a unified approach. Health Aff. 2005; 24: 9-17.
- **El Dib R, Atallah A, Andriolo R.** Mapping the Cochrane evidence for decision making in health care. J Eval Clin Pract. 2007; 13: 689-92.
- **Elstein A.** On the origins and development of evidence-based medicine and medical decision making. Inflamm Res. 2004; 53: 184-9.
- **Friedman L, Furberg C, DeMets D.** Fundamentals of clinical trials, 3rd ed. St. Louis: Mosby; 1996.
- **Goldstein L.** Understanding Medical Statistics. London: William Heinemann Medical Books Limited; 1983.

– **Gopen G.** The Common Sense of Writing: Teaching Writing from the Reader's Perspective; 1990.

– **Greenhalgh T, Donald A.** Evidence based healthcare work-book understanding research. London: BMJ Publishing; 2000.

– **Greenhalgh T.** How to read a paper: the basics of evidence-based medicine. Wiley-Blackwell; 2010.

– **Guyatt G, Rennie D.** Users guides to the medical literature-a manual for evidence based clinical practice by the Evidence-Based Medicine Working Group Chicago, USA: AMA Press; 2001: 356-357.

– **Guyatt G.** Evidence-based medicine. ACP Journal Club. 1991; A18.

– **Hulley S, Newman T, Curnmings S.** Getting started: The anatomy and physiology of clinical research. In: Hulley S, Curnmings S, eds. Designing Clinical Research. Baltimore: Wlliams and Wilkins; 2001.

– **Knapp R, Miller M.** Clinical Epidemiology and Biostatistics. Pennsylvania: Harwal Publishing Company; 1992.

– **Koonce T, Giuse N, Todd P.** Evidence-based databases versus primary medical literature: an in-house investigation on their optimal use. J Med Libr Assoc. 2004; 92: 407-11.

– **Lang T, Secic M.** How to report statistics in medicine. Philadelphia, PA: American College of Physicians; 1997.

– **Moiulsky H.** Intuitive Biostatistics. New York: Oxford University Press; 1995.

– **Nobre M, Bernardo W, Jatene F.** Evidence based clinical practice. Part 1 -- well-structured clinical questions. Rev Assoc Med Bras. 2003; 49: 445-9.

– **Norman G, Streiner D.** Biostatistics. The bare essentials. Missouri, USA: Mosby Year Book Inc; 1994.

- **Pocock S.** Current issues in the design and interpretation of clinical trials. Br Med J. 1985: 296: 39-42.

- **Sackett D, Haynes R, Gyatt G, Tugwell P.** Clinical epidemiology. A basic science for clinical medicine, 2nd ed. Boston: Little, Brown and Company; 1991.

- **Sackett D, Richardson W, Rosenberg W, Haynes R.** Evidence based medicine: How to practice and teach Evidence based medicine, 2nd ed. New: York Churchill Livingstone; 2000.

- **Smith R.** The trouble with medical journals. London: Royal society of Medicine Press; 2006.

- **Straus S, Richardson W, Glasziou P, Haynes R.** Evidence based medicine: How to practice and teach Evidence based medicine. 3rd ed. New York- Elsevier/Churchill Livingstone; 2005.

- **Swinscow T.** Statistics at square one, 9th ed. London British Medical Association; 1994.

- **The Evidence-Based Medicine Working Group.** In Guyatt G, Rennie D, eds. Users' guides to the medical literature. Essentials of evidence based clinical practice. Chicago, IL: AMA Press; 2002.

- **Timmermans S, Mauck A.** The promises and pitfalls of evidence-based medicine. Health Aff. 2005; 24: 18-28.

- **U.S. Preventive Services Task Force.** Guide to clinical preventive services: report of the U.S. Preventive Services Task Force: DIANE Publishing; 1989.

- **World Health Organization.** Handbook for good clinical research practice (GCP): guidance for implementation. Geneva, Switzerland: WHO; 2005.

www.ingramcontent.com/pod-product-compliance
Lightning Source LLC
Chambersburg PA
CBHW051337170526
45166CB00002B/849